SOUL STORIES
OF HEALING

SOUL STORIES
OF HEALING

REIKI STORIES TO INSPIRE YOU

Amy L. Govoni, MSN, RN, RMT

iUniverse LLC
Bloomington

iUniverse books may be ordered through booksellers or by contacting:

iUniverse LLC
1663 Liberty Drive
Bloomington, IN 47403
www.iuniverse.com
1-800-Authors (1-800-288-4677)

ISBN: 978-1-4917-1290-0 (sc)
ISBN: 978-1-4917-1292-4 (hc)
ISBN: 978-1-4917-1291-7 (e)

Printed in the United States of America.

iUniverse rev. date: 11/12/2013

CONTENTS

ACKNOWLEDGEMENTS

Many thanks to all my friends who supported me in so many ways in this book journey! To my family, human and cat, who helped me with tech support, a lot, and loved me every day, I could not have completed this without your understanding! For all of you in my research study and in my world who offered pictures and stories that are close to their hearts, I am so grateful. My editorial friends, many, many thanks! A million hugs to each of you!

PREFACE

Being happy is the cornerstone of all that you are! Nothing is more important than that you feel good. And you have absolute and utter control about that because you can choose the thought that makes you worry or the thought that makes you happy; the things that thrill you, or the things that worry you. You have the choice in every moment. Abraham, *The Science of Deliberate Creation*

I have had many experiences practicing as a nurse for 39 years, working in almost every type of health care setting there is. My specialty as a Board Certified Psychiatric/Mental Health Clinical Nurse Specialist lead me to seek something more for myself and my clients. Reiki became a wonderful tool to add to my practice. I became a Reiki Master Teacher over 15 years ago, practicing and teaching Reiki to individuals and groups. Within these pages are many of my stories as a nurse and a Reiki practitioner. Others are from fellow nurses and those in health care, some of which were part of a research study I conducted on Reiki and Registered Nurses. Some are those moments in life that change its course forever. Each story is filled with heart and lessons learned. Read and immerse yourself in the stories of hope, laughter, joy and change!

"Gratitude is a twofold love—love coming to visit us, and love running out to greet a welcome guest." Henry Van Dyke

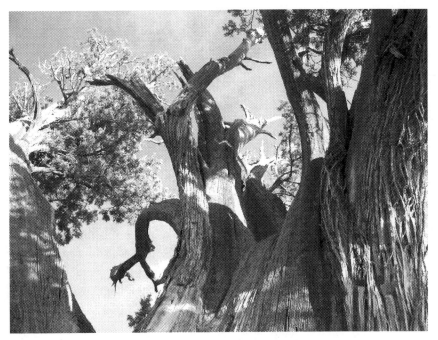

By Amy Govoni

INTRODUCTION

> Every story in our life happens in a way that will never happen
> in exactly the same way again. Details of larger truths played
> out in the personal space of our lives become the essence of our
> unique expressions of our truth. Jack Ricchiuto, *The Stories that
> Connect Us.*

What makes our lives change course? How do we know when life looks
different to us? Why are stories important? These stories we share as
nurses and healers gives us a platform for viewing life. Our stories bind
us together, allow us to learn from each other and allow the wonderful
positive energy to flow to others. Some experiences touched our soul.
Stories are drawn from our raw impressions and beliefs of our life
powerful enough to inspire change or keep us the same. We are our
stories. Learning how to create what your soul treasures is a role of our
life. Here is a place for some of those healing moments that one never
forgets. Each story is unique in its message and heart felt energy that
you will feel, too. Stories share our experiences that have touched our
soul. They are drawn from our raw impressions and beliefs of our life.
Many are powerful enough to inspire change or keep us the same. For
we *are* our stories which connect us to each other. And nurses have more
stories than any book can hold!

The stories are a testament to making a difference in others' lives,
especially for nurses. As nurse angels to some, family to others, and
unforgettable participants in the most terrifying and memorable events
of everyone's lives, nurses have lots of stories! They are privileged to be
part of our most private of moments. But what are *their* most memorable
stories? How did they feel and respond when you were at your lowest or
highest points in life, or crossing over to the other side? They are there
through all of those experiences with stories of strength, compassion,

heartbreak, joy and sadness; heartfelt moments that impacted each of them for life. Some days we ourselves as nurses aren't even sure if what we are doing is worth the effort. Then there is that one moment in time that is frozen forever and lives on in our stories to fortify us on our journey. The days are sometimes long and frustrating, but our stories of healing sustain us. They help us move on to the next person with love, respect, gentleness, joy and humanness. Our stories allow us to continue in our healing practice in whatever form that may take including spiritual peace and contentment.

> You need to claim the events of your life to make yourself yours . . . when you truly possess all you have been, which may take some time, you are fierce with reality." Florida Scott-Maxwell, *The Measure of My Days*

As a Reiki Master Teacher and practitioner, I have heard and experienced many stories involving Reiki. They are powerful in their joyful and healing messages. Reiki is an old Japanese healing practice growing in popularity involving energy work whereby practitioners channel universal energy through their hands to the people they are working on. There is a growing body of scientific study for energy healing practices including Reiki. The National Institutes of Health has funded research for further clinical trials at major scientific centers (http://nccam.nih. gov/health/reiki/introdution.htm.) Clients typically feel warm and relaxed. Dr. Oz has made it a household word and many prominent hospitals in the United States have incorporated it into their offerings for patients and staff. The International Association of Reiki Professionals (IARP) joins 50 countries to work together to give Reiki a strong and wide reaching healing effect throughout the world (www.iarp.org). If you haven't tried it, this will give you a taste of the experience. In America, William Rand and the Reiki Organization, has educated thousands and provides a national forum for educational materials about Reiki and its impact on health (www.reiki.org).

Reiki resources have grown tremendously in the past ten years. Books can be found in any book store or library, with wide spread materials on the web. If interested in becoming certified in Reiki, there are 3 levels of certification, Reiki I, II and Reiki Master Teacher. When seeking instruction, make sure the practitioner is certified at the Reiki Master Teacher level. (See the end of the book for resources on Reiki.)

> "Humans are bio crystalline beings. We can re pattern any corrupted cells of our body to become loving, healthy, joyous, prosperous and peaceful; which is our original Divine blueprint." Laurelle Shanti Gaia

Some of the stories are about animals, or animal angels as I like to call them. These wonderful creatures totally get us as no one else does. They totally accept us when no one else could. And they are there to guide us in our journey of life! Remember your first pet? That one that understood your unspoken needs and wants that even your closest friends didn't? Yes, these animal stories will remind you to reflect on those wonderful partners with fur, fins or scales in your life. Unconditional love with fur . . .

> "Be thankful for what you have; you'll end up having more. If you concentrate on what you don't have, you will never, ever have enough." Oprah Winfrey

When you read these Soul Stories, think of your own—how similar are they? Can you learn from that story? Or is the energy it projects just what you need right now? You can open the book anywhere and see what speaks to you, or you can read it in order. There is no right or wrong way to experience them. You will know what is right for you. The stories have some general themes the affect our lives: animals, nursing experiences, children, life and death, Reiki, and human experience.

So settle in, open this book and immerse yourself in the love, light and joy of wonderful positive energy within these stories. If this book could come with a fireplace and blanket, it would! If you are a nurse or in health care and are having a tough time right now with the challenges that face you, read the stories. Has life just seemed a bit too shallow lately? Read the stories. Each story has lessons learned, with pictures that speak to us without words and quotes that sharpen our messages. Live the life we want versus the life we think we must live. Many thanks to all the research participants and friends who have graciously offered their stories for this publication. Due to confidentiality restraints, no names have been attributed to any stories and those used in the stories are fictitious. Let me know if you have your own stories. Send them to: amygovoni@gmail.com Looking forward to hearing from you all!

> "Fear, like joy, usually means that you're exactly where you should be, learning what you're ready to learn, about to become more than who you were." Michael Dooley

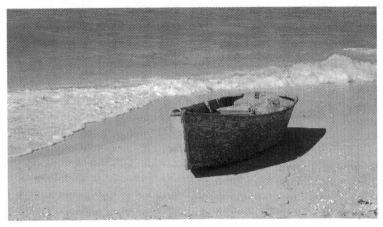

By Michael Bozeman

1

NEVER FORGETTING THAT PERSON

"The effects of kindness are not always seen immediately. Sometimes it takes years until your kindness will pay off. Sometimes you never see the fruits of your labors, but they are there, deep inside of the soul of the one you touched." Dan Kelly

After nearly 40 years as a registered nurse I can recall many memorable patients. Regardless of the specific circumstances as to why I think that I have remembered them, such as my first patient who died or my first patient who's heart stopped beating, I truly believe that the memories are so deeply embedded in my mind because the interactions with these patients have made me a better nurse. Long before shortened lengths of stays and before the word homelessness came into my vocabulary I met Augie.

Augie, as we all fondly called him, was a hobo. At the time, in the early 70s, being a hobo was romanticized in song, in poems, and in television and movies. They were a band of vagabonds that hitchhiked or rode the rails across the country, hopping on and off trains as the will so moved them or as such time that they disembarked courtesy of the conductor of the train. They worked at odd jobs and allowed kind people to lend them a dollar or feed them a meal.

He came to the neuro intensive care unit from a local railroad yard. He had a brain contusion and decreased level of consciousness, the cause of which was never known. He was nonverbal and did not regain full consciousness for some time. That was not what made him so memorable.

I was on duty the evening he was admitted. He had identification, but no evidence of any family or friends. No one called and no one visited. If he had family, they were estranged. If he had friends, they were long gone. No pictures or telling tattoos. What struck us all so clearly was how unkempt he was! He had very long, dirty, matted, and smelly hair! His beard was a match for the hair. His fingernails were crusty, long and in terrible condition. His toenails matched. Although the initial plan was to stabilize him and decrease the pressure in his brain, our hidden agenda was to clean him up. Once it was very evident that he was getting better, not in leaps and bounds, but at a snail's pace, it was time for his nurses to take action.

It was a small group process, for when one of us was off duty another nurse took over. First we shampooed, several times as I recall. I then asked the neurosurgeon if I could start trimming his hair and beard. Of course, he said yes. The group of us then started on his feet and hands. I soaked them and softened them. We took turns filing away at the fingernails and sought out a podiatrist to take care of the feet. Over time Augie looked better and slowly he began to recover. He was able to eat, sit in a chair, and be transferred to the care of a family physician. He began to talk but had no recollection of his injury. He had been admitted in the fall and was there through Christmas and even into the early spring. He looked forward to his 'girls' coming to visit and for the treats we brought him. Nothing big but things he loved like grooming items and homemade cookies. He had a sparkling smile. He would hug us and we would let him. By early spring, it was time for the social worker to find Augie a place to go. They settled for a bed in a county home. We all said our goodbyes. Augie was out of sight but not out of our minds and our hearts.

The day after his discharge, the family physician came to the unit and told us that "Augie" had died. I remember his words so clearly. "I think he died of a broken heart. You all truly cared for him and he loved you. It is the only explanation as to why he died." Caring for Augie was the right thing to do. We cared for him as a patient. We cared for him because he was a kind soul. From this experience I learned the connection between the body, mind, and spirit. His unexplained death attributed by the physician to a 'broken heart' was a lesson learned. Also, the fact that this physician recognized the contribution nursing made to this patient's care and recovery, was also a very special lesson for me. For the physician to seek us out to tell us in person helped me realize how very important we are in our patients' lives.

I was probably in my early 20s as I graduated from nursing school when I was 20, too young to deal with the realities of nursing. I was so taken by the kindness and caring of the family physician, that I became his patient until I moved away from Cleveland. The doctor himself was so kind and caring . . . he saw Augie as a real human being as well. It was a great experience.

Lesson learned: Always treat others as human beings, no matter what their background and where they have come from. We are all human beings worthy of love and respect. We are put in different situations as healers, young and old, for a reason. Nothing is by chance. Synchronicities are everywhere. We just need to be open to them and listen to their messages.

> I have never met a person whose greatest need was anything other than real, unconditional love. You can find it in a simple act of kindness toward someone who needs help. There is no mistaking love. You feel it in your heart. It is the common fiber of life, the flame that heals our soul, energizes our spirit and supplies passion to our lives. Elizabeth Kubler-Ross

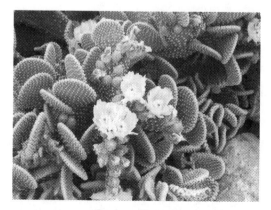

By Amy Govoni

2

MIRACLE OF A HORSE

"The real reason animals don't talk is because they understand
so much." Unknown author

This is a story of a very important horse, unlike any of the many horses I
have had in my life. His name was Mel. He was a constant in my life for
many years. Through all of the good times and bad times, he was with
me. Life changes, things come and go, but I always had Mel at my side.

It was around Thanksgiving time when I was diagnosed with stage 3
ovarian cancer. After my surgery I was often weak, and felt drained and
tired. Then came the chemotherapy, which took away every ounce of my
energy. I felt scared. I stayed inside much of the time. When I pushed
myself to walk out to the barn, I would stand next to Mel, and tell him
that I would ride him again one day. Petting his warm body seemed to
heal mine. It was always quiet in the barn, no one but the horses and me.
I would marvel at his power and beauty. After spending time rubbing
my hands over his soft neck, I would feel more in touch with life, as if
embraced by his energy. I could feel his strength filling me with hope.
I made frequent walks out to the barn and reassured Mel that I would
ride him when I was stronger.

After my chemotherapy was over, still feeling quite weak, my husband
helped me up onto Mel's back. I was excited. It felt so familiar, a part of
my old life that I thought I had lost. I had been riding Mel for 20 years.
I rode him through my divorce, I rode him through the death of my
little sister, and now I rode him for the first time after my cancer. I felt
him move in a sluggish fashion and told my husband he was as out of
shape as I was. That was the last time I rode him. He died two days after

I managed to get on him. He took a piece of my heart with him, but left me his strength. I believe he waited for me to get well before he could die.

I think Mel helped me heal. My husband says he died instead of me, allowing me to live. Whatever the event meant, I appreciate the strength he gave me to get through my most difficult times. I think he had a powerful healing spirit that continues to live within me. He will always be with me . . .

Lesson learned: Appreciate the animal angels that we are honored to be touched by. They hold the mysteries of the universe within them and they are willing and able to share them with us. Use them when you can for healing and caring for others. They are ready and willing. Feel and listen to their messages. They are here for us.

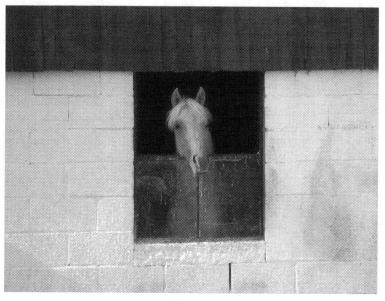

By Margaret Toukonen

5

3

—⁓⁓∘⊙⦁⟿⊙⦁∘⁓⁓—

PARENTS' GIFTS

"If you begin looking at each breath as a blessing, then suddenly
everything in an ordinary life becomes a miracle-delighting in
the colors of the setting sun, feeling the rain on your face or
smelling the amazing fragrance of a single perfect rose." Kirsti
A. Dyer

My Dad was a simple but amazing man . . . a double leg amputee from
World War II. Growing up I thought all dads had wooden legs next to
their beds. It didn't faze me at all, as Dad considered it so normal, he
never made a big deal about it. Imagine, losing your legs while fighting
for our country at 26 years of age with your wife home pregnant with
your first child! When I complain, I think of Dad and then I am ashamed.
It is all in perspective as he never complained, made a fuss about having
no legs, made anyone feel bad about his being different nor did he miss
out on anything in life. He almost could run with those legs. He rode
the famous wooden roller coaster at Euclid Beach Amusement Park near
Cleveland, Ohio, with me and took me to every one of the Cleveland
Indians baseball games when I finally got straight A's and those golden
Indians' tickets! He was romantic to my mom, made everyone laugh and
didn't have a mean bone in his body.

All of this hit me one night as I was working as an RN on a step down
unit. In those days, people actually stayed in the hospital after their major
surgeries. I found a woman with incredible challenges with her parents,
including abuse, neglect and cruelty of unimaginable proportions. I
finally realized how lucky I was. When I came home after my evening
shift and flung myself into my parents' arms, I am sure they thought I
was insane. But that was my moment when I truly realized how lucky

and blessed I was. And I wasn't going to let all that effort from my parents go to waste! I wanted to make sure I passed it on to everyone I could. I still hold that promise close to my heart today even though both my parents are gone. I believe they know . . .

Lesson learned: Appreciate all the gifts your parents give you, especially the ones that last a lifetime. Thank them when they are still on this earth plane. Know they are doing the best they can in this moment in time. Learn from their mistakes and send them love. They were only doing what they think/thought they should do. Framing our childhood and the parents that made it is an adult lesson we all must learn and know how to thrive within. It will help you on your healing path.

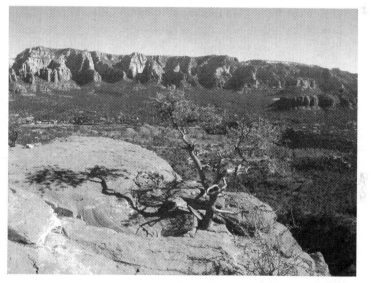

By Amy Govoni

4

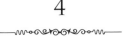

ONE PERSON MAKING A DIFFERENCE

"When we become more fully aware that our success is due in large measure to the loyalty, helpfulness, and encouragement we have received from others, our desire grows to pass on similar gifts. Gratitude spurs us on to prove ourselves worthy of what others have done for us. The spirit of gratitude is a powerful energizer." Wilferd A. Peterson

When I was in my junior year in high school, I found myself taking French in the same class as my sister who was a freshman. Since we had to take two years of Latin when I started high school, this was my first experience with a spoken foreign language. My sister is a very gifted student, who studied very little and always got straight A's. She picked up French very easily, and was light years ahead of me, even though we studied together and conversed back and forth. In class my sister shone brightly with her perfect accent and easy conversation. I have always had to study hard, and work for every grade I got, so this was pretty intimidating.

This did not go unnoticed by our teacher Sr. Rachael. One afternoon after class, she stopped me in the hall and pulled me over to the side to talk. I thought I was in big trouble! She just looked me straight in the eye, and told me not to be intimidated by my sister. I was taken a back, as I didn't know that anyone knew what I was feeling. She then said that I could do anything in life that I wanted to, I had the ability.

These word of encouragement have stayed with me a lifetime. When I have felt uneasy about trying something new or different I remember what Sr. Rachael said that day in the hall. I have been successful in life, and I feel that things may have been different had that brief encountered in the hall of my junior year of high school not happened. It was truly life changing!

Lesson Learned: We never know how our caring practice will effect others and how many years it will effect them. Know that each day these people will feel your energy, your caring touch and carry it with them always. Some will acknowledge this, others will take many years to be open to it. But you will always make an impact . . . make it a good one!

5

REIKI AND MIRACLES

"Have regular hours for work and play; make each day both useful and pleasant, and prove that you understand the worth of time by employing it well. Then youth will be delightful, old age will bring few regrets and life will become a beautiful success."
Louisa May Alcott

One night a friend, an RN who also does Reiki, called me. Her son's friend had been in a 100 mph motorcycle accident. and she asked me to help with his healing. We sent long distance Reiki from our homes to try to get him through the night and then she asked me if I would meet her the next day in the Intensive Care Unit to do Reiki on her son's friend. We went the next day and got the parents' permission to give him Reiki.

We promised to only spend 10 minutes on him so they could visit. He also looked to be about 250 lbs and his face was so swollen that there were no definitive features. He had multiple, serious injuries to so many body systems! As soon as we started the Reiki, the monitors started ringing and wouldn't stop until the nurse adjusted them. Maybe this was energy at work? We started at the head working our way down his body. I concentrated on the left arm that had had surgery because there was still no pulse and they still might have to amputate it. Both my hands had intense pulsing and throbbing from all the damage he had.

That evening I got a call from my friend. Her son went to see him an hour after we left, and the parents told him that 10 minutes after we left, the swelling significantly went down, his blood pressure stabilized for the first time since he came in, he started breathing on his own off the ventilator and they found a pulse in his left arm! We worked on him every day either in person or long distance and he was discharged a month later. The Dr. told him he was 3 months ahead of what would be expected in healing. Being a tall skinny 22 year old male that only weighed about 110 pounds made it even more of a miracle.

Lessons Learned: The impossible becomes possible when we just believe for the highest good when we give to someone without personal need or gain.

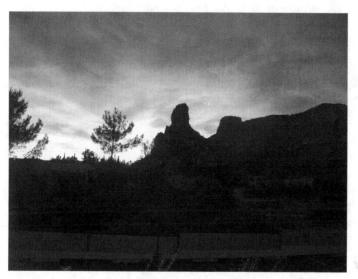

By Amy Govoni

"Time and health are two precious assets that we don't recognize and appreciate until they have been depleted." Unknown

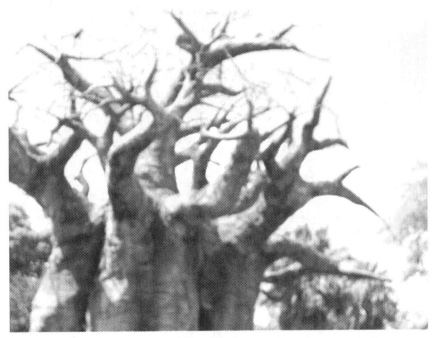

By Amy Govoni

6

REIKI VS. HOPELESSNESS

"Sometimes life is just that . . . a moment in time that we do our best with." Unknown

I worked with an acquaintance of my mother's, a woman diagnosed with the most aggressive type of breast cancer. She was told to get her papers in order and plan her funeral as she would die within 3 months and there was nothing more her oncologist could do for her. She also was dealing with a major loss. Her husband had died prematurely and quite unexpectedly. She came to me with tears dripping down her face, dealing with the double grief of losing her husband suddenly, and then her own devastating cancer diagnosis. She could hardly get on the table, so heavy was she with grief. As I moved my hands over her body, the heart area was completely empty of energy! I could almost feel her broken heart, as my hands felt cold, and empty. She continued to softly cry throughout the treatment, at one point, holding my hand and unable to let go.

After the Reiki treatment, she had a huge emotional release forgiving her husband's death. The tears flowed even more freely, but she had a curious smile on her face. She said it felt like she was truly a new energetic person, which she had not experienced for many years. Though still sad, she knew in that moment she could move on and let go of the awful heaviness and anger surrounding her husband's death.

Further treatments for her breast cancer issues continued. My hands felt energy above and below her breasts was a curious combination of hot, hot energy and cold emptiness. We worked on this for a number of Reiki treatments. She was quite anxious as the date to meet with her oncologist drew near. When she returned to her oncologist, the masses in her breasts that were cancerous were found to be diminished to the point where the oncologist agreed that now radiation and surgery would be helpful.

Her cancer was successfully treated. Today, she not only is alive, but has inherited millions from a woman she worked for after getting ill. What a blessing to be part of that wonderful ending!

Lesson Learned: In our earthly existence, the end may only be the beginning as the plans for our future are not always that clear to us.

7

CHANGING A LIFE WITH REIKI

"Your task is not to seek for love, but merely to seek and find all the barriers within yourself that you have built against it." Rumi

I have been working with a man who was agoraphobic, an abnormal fear of being helpless in an embarrassing or inescapable situation that is characterized especially by the avoidance of open or public places, when he first ventured out to see me. After one year of weekly Reiki he has his own business, has a social life and his primary care physician has cut his psychotropic drugs in half. He has more focus and clarity dealing with his daily problems and life. He has made an amazing recovery and continues to see me for tune-ups.

Lesson Learned: When the impossible becomes possible, our messages become clear to us. We just need to pay attention and listen.

8

LISTENING TO ONE'S INUITIVE VOICE

"Celebrate what you want to see more of." Tom Peters

The first time I "intuited" the area of concern in a client was the most amazing and humbling experience. For me, that means that my inner voice gave me a message and I listened to it. My hands were on a woman's upper abdomen, and I had the very clear message to move them to her lower abdomen. I began to feel pain in my body in the left lower quadrant. I asked her if there was anything of concern in this area. She seemed amazed and said this is where she had colon cancer and surgery.

Lesson Learned: It is always amazing when we listen to our inner voice and the outcome becomes so clear to us! Now listening more becomes second nature and the messages become clearer. Our biggest challenge is to get out of our own way.

9

SHARING THE MESSAGE

"If you believe in what you are doing, then let nothing hold you up in your work. Much of the best work of the world has been done against seeming impossibilities. The thing is to get the work done." Dale Carnegie

A very physically healthy young woman came to me for emotional relief because she had lost 3 significant people in her life over the past six months and was feeling anger, depression, and grief over the deaths. The most significant was the loss of her mother who died unexpectedly 2 months before and she was having a very difficult time coping with that loss in particular. During her Reiki treatment I kept seeing the color purple. While some Reiki practitioners see colors, it is not typical for me and I had the strong feeling her mother was somehow "offering her the color purple." I can't even begin to explain that but it was an intuitive knowledge that came to me that I have learned over the years to trust. I could also feel that my client needed to do some very intense physical activity to help work out the grief and resulting anger I felt energetically trapped in her body.

After the treatment, I suggested some type of healthy vigorous activity and she said she had just seen a Tao Bo class she wanted to take. Her treatment confirmed her decision to sign up. But more significantly she was stunned when I told her it might be good to put things of purple around her room, include in her clothing accessories. I told her I didn't know exactly why but I intuitively felt during her treatment that things of this color would somehow signify a loving connection with her mom that is beyond death. She started crying and saying her mom's favorite color was purple. Both the client and I felt a deep sense of the profound after the treatment.

Lessons Learned: Listening to ourselves is sometimes the hardest lesson to learn and trust. Messages and synchronicities become daily as our minds open to the possibilities. The Chakra colors, those of our energy wheels, may give us messages about what we are trying to grapple with.

10

———〜〜◦◦◦◦◦◦◦〜〜———

THE POWER OF REIKI

"At times our own light goes out and is rekindled by a spark from another person. Each of us has cause to think with deep gratitude of those who have lighted the flame within us." Albert Schweitzer

I have made a difference to many patients by giving them Reiki, from lowering blood pressure when the IV medications weren't working, to increasing bowel activity that had slowed down after surgery. Many times I use energy work to relieve pain. This happens frequently when the pain medications aren't working well enough for the patient to be comfortable. Their pain relief from my work always amazes me. It's like I could stay there, hands-on, indefinitely because it means so much to them.

Lesson learned: Pain relief is a wonderful gift for the person receiving and the one giving. It provides us with the opportunity to share with others without the burden of pain to weigh us down. The lessons of pain, however, are many. What is your lesson from your pain or those you care for?

Intuitive Messages from the Universe, angels and ascended masters beyond our earth realm of understanding that are received by the practitioner are open to interpretation from the healer and the client. Mostly, the symbolic nature of intuitive messages allow the healer to present questions and possibilities in the most positive way. With practice, the symbolic nature of the messages becomes easier to interpret and share with the client. The clients are the ones that will know and find their own meanings to the messages, sometimes immediately but often days, weeks or months later.

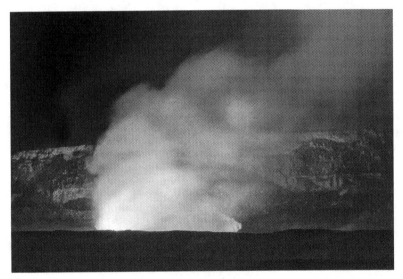

By Bill Brodnick

11

——⟨ornamental divider⟩——

STAYING CENTERED THROUGH LOSS AND GRIEF

"If you begin looking at each breath as a blessing, then suddenly everything in an ordinary life becomes a miracle-delighting in the colors of the setting sun, feeling the rain on your face or smelling the amazing fragrance of a single perfect rose." Kirsti A. Dyer

To journey through life is to expect ups and downs, for the road is bumpy. When I think about experiences that have caused me to stop and learn from the moment, there are many. These moments make us who we are and who we will be. I would like to take a few moments to share a moment.

When my son was 29 years old he committed suicide. Any person who had lost a child under any circumstance understands the depth of the pain that you carry in your heart. The journey through grief is long and dark many times feeling that you will never be able to smile, laugh or love again.

It has been five years now since his passing. A number of his friends have stayed in contact with me. Often they have warmed my heart with stories of their times together. These stories provided me peace knowing that my son made a difference in their lives and they still remember with love. However, the emptiness in my heart remains.

Which brings me to my moment of wonderment. My daughter and I vacation together every other year. During this vacation she convinced me that it would be an adventure to explore the southwest in August. I am not a hot weather person and the desert during that time of year did not appeal to my sense of adventure, but we ended up going.

Since my son died I have had the opportunity to enjoy many breath taking moments with my remaining son and daughter. I have visited my son in St. Croix where he lives and experiences sunset, rain storms and the quick to appear rainbows that follow the storms. When my daughter and I traveled in the Dakota's at dusk we watched a herd of buffalo walking by the field and roadside releasing the fragrance of clover as they continued on their journey. But nothing could ever prepare me for the experience that was found at the north rim of the Grand Canyon.

As I approached the overlook to the canyon, I was hot and tired. A storm was in the distance and the thunder echoed through the canyon. My daughter went ahead of me as I walked slowly through a gravel path which would lead me to the canyon. I noticed tall bushes on each side of the walkway and as the wind blew I caught a fragrance that warmed my being. I stopped to explore these bushes to see what could possibly be providing such a sweet smell. I quickly found the source. The bushes were roses in full bloom. I surrounded myself with the bushes smelling the most beautiful fragrance I had every experienced in my life. At that moment I found comfort, peace, warmth and understanding. No matter how difficult my journey has been I will always be able to remember the fragrance that helped me to understand my path. That moment will be carried in my heart forever. When sad memories flood my soul, I will remember the peace found in the desert rose. I now understand what Sting was teaching when he sang, "this desert flower, this rare perfume, the sweet intoxication of life."

Lesson learned: So many lessons . . . soul lessons for the heart when it seems to be breaking apart.

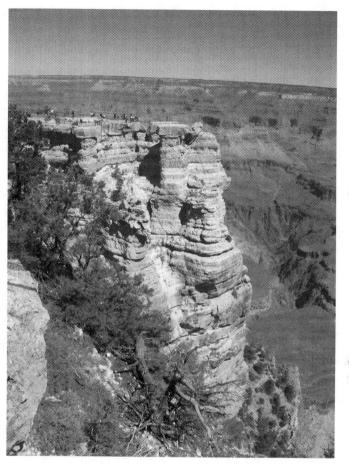

By Amy Govoni

12

A Mother's Gratitude

"The grand essentials of happiness are: Something to do, something to love and something to hope for." Allan K. Chalmers

I was working on a baby who had an IV (intravenous needle) in her hand. She was so small! The IV had infiltrated, allowing fluid from the bag to flow into the baby's hand tissues where it should not have gone. This made the baby's hand very swollen, cold and white. The mom was so worried and didn't know how to comfort her crying child. I asked if I could give the baby some Reiki to comfort her. She agreed and I gave the baby's hand Reiki for about 15 mins. The fluid seeped out of the tissues, which allowed the swelling to go down. The skin became warm and pink! There was no permanent tissue damage! Wow! The mom was so grateful as was I! The baby smiled! I'll never forget the baby's/mom's smile . . .

Lesson learned: We are filled with wonder by the relief and joy we can provide through Reiki. We ache as mothers and caregivers when we feel the pain of a child's experience. Knowing we can provide some relief is a blessing.

13

―――ᴡᴡᴏᴏᴏᴏᴏ⊙ᴏᴏᴡᴡ―――

REIKI AS A GIFT FOR SELF

"We delight in the beauty of the butterfly, but rarely admit the changes it has gone through to achieve that beauty." Maya Angelou

I lost my husband of 31 years last May. It was long and painful. Performing Reiki on myself helped me calm and center. I needed this so much in those early days! What a gift to myself! It warmed my life at a time where I was so overcome with grief and loss. I am so thankful . . .

Lesson learned: Be good to oneself; remember to give ourselves the gifts we give others. Caring for ourselves is usually last on our list. Self care is one of the most important things we can do as caregivers and healers for ourselves. It lifts us up, gives us strength and courage to move on to heal another day. Without it, our spirit shrivels and dies. Sometimes, this lack of care for ourselves forces us to stop healing. We need to make ourselves as important as those we care for.

14

—⁓⦿⦾⦿⦾⁓—

PHYSICAL PAIN RELIEF

"Be glad of life because it gives you the chance to love and to work and to play and to look up at the stars." Henry Van Dyke

I gave a cancer patient Reiki who was in excruciating pain when I was a nursing student. Just being a student, I had my doubts about what I could do to help her. Her daughter was also a Reiki practitioner. She was young, only in her 30's. The patient held my hand tightly, and would not let me leave her side. She told the other nurses, that she will not let them do anything unless I was in the room, holding her hand. I stayed with her until she fell asleep. She was in much less pain when I left that day.

Lesson learned: You are never "only a student, mother, father or child"! These don't weaken your power to comfort, heal and provide relief to those you touch. Acknowledging your healing potential is the first step. Our impact is far reaching.

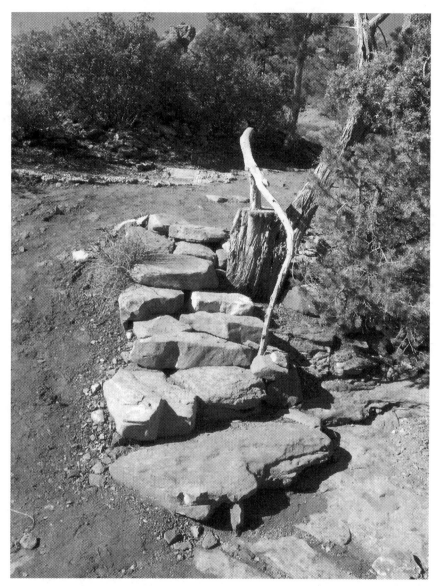

By Amy Govoni

15

PERSONAL INTUITIVE MESSAGES

"You cannot live a perfect day without doing something for someone who will never be able to repay you." John Wooden

One person who was extremely skeptical of all things "alternative", whom I had expected to come in with a closed mind and spirit, actually had an experience of seeing images during her Reiki session. The images were clear and left her speechless. Each image had a special meaning to her. She was initially frightened and surprised. We talked through each message which left her open to more possibilities in her life. Feeling that she needed to leave an abusive relationship for a long time, this gave her the support and courage to follow through. She's a changed woman now with a much more open mind and healthier body. It was such a pleasure to see her putting herself first.

Lesson learned: Don't anticipate or make a judgment about how the person you are treating may experience your interaction. You aren't in control of that anyway. The Universe is. They will experience what they need to. As long as they are open, there will be a positive outcome.

16

—⁓⁓⦿⟋⟍⦿⟍⦿⟋⦿⟋⟍⦿⟋⟍⦿⟋⦿—

TRUSTING OUR INNER VOICES

"We are not human beings on a spiritual journey. We are spiritual beings on a human journey." Dr. Stephen Covey

The first time I "intuited" the area of concern in a client was the most amazing and humbling experience. For me, that means that my inner voice gave me a message and I listened to it. My hands were on a woman's upper abdomen and I had the very clear message to move them to her lower abdomen. I began to feel pain in my body in the left lower quadrant. I asked her if there was anything of concern in this area. She seemed amazed and said this is where she had colon cancer and surgery.

Lesson Learned: It is always amazing when we listen to our inner voice and the outcome becomes so clear to us! Now listening more becomes second nature and the messages become clearer. Our biggest challenge is to get out of our own way.

17

BELIEVING AND DISCOVERING MEANING

"The only limits in your life are those that you set yourself."
Unknown

A woman came to me for an Intuitive Reiki session. It was filled with alot of Reiki energy for her intention of stress reduction. Her intuitive messages, however, were not very clear in meaning to either the client or the healer. One in particular was repeated over and over. It was two capital letters backwards. Neither of us could decipher their meaning. The client left refreshed and relaxed from the session, but puzzled as to the letters' meanings. One month later she called me with great excitement. She said, "Do you remember the letters backwards?" Of course I did, as it was such a clear message which neither of us could decode. "Well, I have figured it out! Remember my young son who was having so many difficulties at school? He was diagnosed with dyslexia! And the letters? They are his initials, backwards!" We were both speechless at this wonderful news! If only all messages could be this clear at the time they are received!

Lesson learned: Don't doubt yourself if the intuitive message is confusing to you. Know that there is a reason it was sent to the client, and the client will be able to figure it out. You can be supportive and give them ideas of the possibilities, but you are not the one that knows the answer.

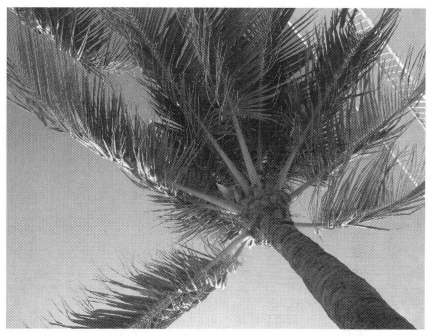

By Amy Govoni

18

—⁓⁓◦◦◦◦⁓⁓—

ANGELS AND PAIN

"Remember, we are all affecting the world every moment, whether we mean to or not. Our actions and states of mind matter because we are so deeply interconnected. Working on our own consciousness is the most important thing that we are doing at any moment, and being love is the supreme creative act." Ram Dass

A client in severe pain for many, many years reported to me that with only one Reiki treatment, her pain was completely gone for eight weeks, and her ability to walk was greatly improved. As powerful as Reiki is, even I was stunned, given her health condition. I thank the angels for their guidance on that! From my view, every Reiki session is unique. I too, feel feedback from all of my senses—primarily from my sense of touch, but I often get feedback from my vision or "inner ears". I only let them give some of this feedback if I feel it is urgent or necessary for healing.

Lesson Learned: Listening to that voice that only you can hear can provide much support in caring for our fellow humans here on earth. It is that inner voice that allows us to truly treat the whole person. How we interpret that voice is a life long lesson in listening.

19

——∿∘◦◦◦◦∿——

HEALING WOUNDS

"Nothing of great value in life comes easily. The things of highest
value sometimes come hard. The gold that has the greatest value lies
deepest in the earth, as do the diamonds." Norman Vincent Peale

One client I worked on had a very severe injury to his skin and several
layer of tissues—however, I was not aware of it at the time I was called
to give him Reiki, as it was under his clothing. I only knew he had a
problem and was in pain. I did a full body treatment, scanning for
issues by placing my hands a few inches over his body. Only afterward
did he tell me and show me the damage. He did not feel any pain after
the treatment, and 24 hours later, this oozy, nasty looking wound was
scaling over and drying. Healing was taking place quickly!

Lesson learned: We don't need lots of information prior to giving a Reiki
treatment. Only openness to what will be for the highest good of the
client is needed along with our own grounded experiences.

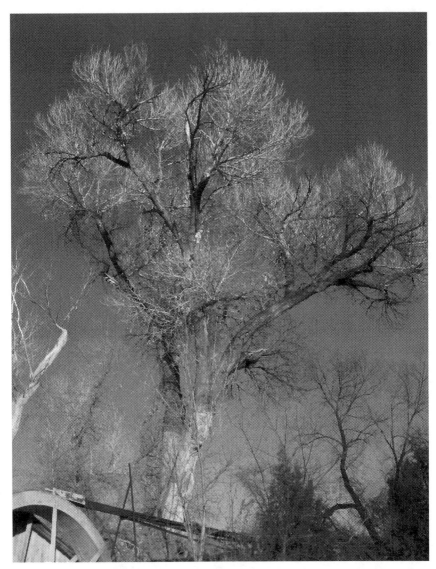

By Amy Govoni

20

REIKI WITH AN AUDIENCE

"Try not to resist the changes that come your way. Instead let life move through you. And do not worry that your life is turning upside down. How do you know that the side you are used to is better than the one to come?" Rumi

I was part of a presentation / panel discussion about Reiki and Healing Touch for an organization that provides services and support to people with cancer diagnosis. There were approximately 35 people attending, none of whom I knew. As part of my presentation on Reiki, I opened my hands out to the audience and told them that I was offering Reiki energy to all of them at that moment. My purpose in doing this was to show them how simple it is to send this energy to anyone who wants to accept it. Then I went on with my talk.

A few weeks later, I met one of the participants who came for my individual Reiki sessions. He has a diagnosis of kidney cancer with metastasis which he had know about for about 6 years. He had been having left shoulder pain for a while, seeing his doctor regularly, worrying that the cancer had spread further. He was in the audience that day for my presentation. He said that after I offered Reiki to everyone his shoulder pain went away and had not come back. This happened about a year ago. This man comes to see me on a regular basis and when I see him, he mentions this group event. He feels that Reiki healed the pain in his shoulder at that moment at that presentation!

Lesson learned: We do not know how our gifts can help others; just remember to keep giving them. What a wonderful gift to offer to others!

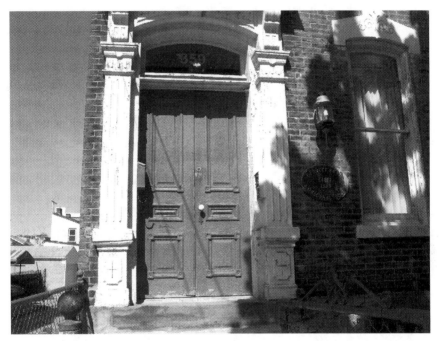

By Amy Govoni

Distance Reiki is a technique that is learned in the Reiki II certification. Using a specific Japanese Distance Symbol, one is able to send Reiki anywhere it is needed. There are a couple of ways to do this. The healer can set a specific time for the Reiki to be sent, or, they can send it at anytime. The practitioner prepares as for an in person session, draws the Distance Symbol and then raises their hands to send the Reiki in the general direction it should go. The only important rule is that the person must be open to and want the Reiki to be sent. This is a wonderful technique to use for anyone who is not with you that is in need of Reiki help.

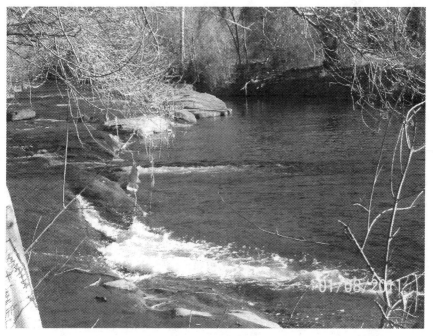

By Amy Govoni

21

SENDING REIKI FOR PAIN RELIEF

"From the standpoint of daily life, however, there is one thing we do know: that we are here for the sake of each other – above all for those upon whose smile and well-being our own happiness depends, and also for the countless unknown souls with whose fate we are connected by a bond of sympathy. Many times a day I realize how much my own outer and inner life is built upon the labors of my fellow men, both living and dead, and how earnestly I must exert myself in order to give in return as much as I have received." Albert Einstein

A colleague was asking for Reiki for hip pain before I left work that night. I asked if I could give her some distantly because I needed to leave. She said fine. It was about 11 p.m. And I started to do Reiki from her head down. I felt a lot of energy when I was doing her head area, never getting to the hip before I fell asleep. The next day, I told her that I did a treatment before falling asleep and that I didn't get past her head, which was full of energy. She told me that she had an argument with her husband that evening about her being late getting home, right about the time I was doing the Reiki treatment. She wasn't surprised about her "headiness," but what did surprise her was that her hip pain was gone!

Lesson learned: Distant Reiki is easy and effortless. Being able to offer energy to those who aren't with you is unbelievably affirming. We are healers in so many ways. Believe in one's ability to provide relief to others and always be ready for the unexpected, welcoming it with gratitude and joy! This is especially true when one doubts oneself and one's impact on others. As healers we have the ability to share our gifts with those that need it most. We don't have to think about it. We do it.

22

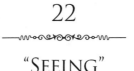

"Seeing"

"Piglet noticed that even though he had a Very Small Heart,
it could hold a rather large amount of Gratitude." A.A. Milne

I was in Reiki class, and we were practicing Long Distance Reiki. I was sending Reiki to the Middle East conflict, which was escalated at the time. I saw Jesus on the other side of the ball I was holding, also holding a ball of light. When I shared the story with my teacher, she said "I am glad he is on the job." It was an amazing experience for me. I have also had many more experiences like this one.

Lesson Learned: Belief systems are powerful for ourselves and those we care for. Allowing ourselves and our clients the openness to whatever belief system they have to help them heal during Reiki frees all of us of our preconceived notions of healing and religion. Those beliefs don't have to be limiting. They can be freeing!

23

SENDING REIKI TO DECREASE PAIN

"Learn from the past, set vivid, detailed goals for the future, and live in the only moment of time over which you have any control: now." Denis Waitley

I was sending Reiki from a distance to a fellow non-believing nurse. Her issue was pain when walking on her right foot. For some reason I was drawn to her left hip. So I directed the energy to the hip. After the long distance session, I asked if there was anything wrong because I felt a tremendous surge of energy around her left hip. Apparently she had injured it the day before and I had no knowledge of this. She stated that she was in a lot of pain but from the hip she injured. The next day she called me and told me the pain was gone! She spoke in wonder, and was very thankful for my treatment. :)

Lesson learned: Trust oneself when that little voice tells you to do something you never thought you would do. The messages from the Universe are usually right! We just need to listen to them and know they are tools in our healing journey. Sometimes they give us warnings of what lies ahead and gives us a chance to alter the course of the path for others and ourselves.

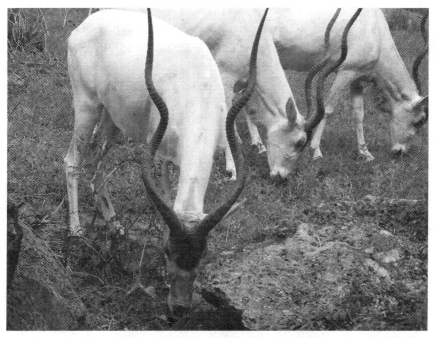

By Amy Govoni

24

—∿∿⚬⚬〰⚬⚬∿∿—

VISUALIZING WOUNDS

"People usually consider walking on water or in thin air a miracle but I think the real miracle is not to walk either on water or in thin air, but to walk on earth. Every day we are engaged in a miracle which we don't even recognize: a blue sky, white clouds, green leaves, the black, curious eyes of a child—our own two eyes. All is a miracle." Thich Nhat Han

I was offering Reiki to a friend who gave a very strong verbal intention at the beginning of the session to cleanse herself. As I began to offer Reiki to her throat chakra, she told me that she could visualize a woman who was sweeping down her chakra, moving energy away from her—energy that no longer served her highest good. Suddenly, she felt that she had a blockage in her throat area and upper right chest. She described it as dark, sticky, and immovable. I began to energetically drain the area for her. She said that the area was like a very deep dark cavern or cave. Like a dark wound. As I continued to drain this area, she described a change in the wound. It became redder and inflamed. Then she felt scared and asked me several times not to leave her. She felt as though there was going to be an explosion. I repeatedly reassured her that she was in a safe and protected place. Then the wound became filled with pink healthy tissue according to her descriptions. I continued the energetic drain and told her to tell me when the draining was completed. Eventually she felt that I could stop draining and I began to offer Reiki healing to the area. She said that the blockage was mostly gone, that there was just some light gray color lingering around her neck.

I have worked with this woman a number of times and her response to Reiki has always been profound, intense, and very visual. What was so interesting about this session was that this etheric blockage seemed to go thru the actual stages of wound healing that we see in the physical body. Her descriptions were colorful and exact.

Lesson learned: Sometimes the lesson is not for us as healers, but for those healed.

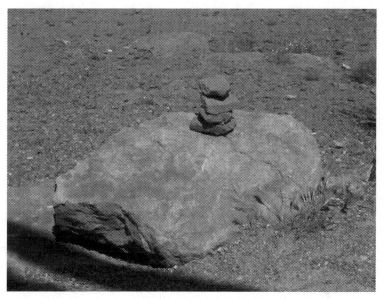

By Amy Govoni

25

NURSES MAKING A DIFFERENCE

"The world is a great mirror. It reflects back to you what you are. If you are loving, if you are friendly, if you are helpful, the world will prove loving and friendly and helpful to you. The world is what you are." Thomas Dreier

Do nurses make a difference? I was brought up in the fifties. My mother and her nurse friends used to sit around our kitchen table and discuss how they were going to make a difference at an inner city hospital in Chicago. 5 nurses who drank dark black coffee and smoked menthol cigarettes nonstop, attempting to make a difference. I would sit in the doorway of the kitchen after school as a young girl and listen attentively to "their plan." Why were babies born with "birth defects" or low birth weights put in room alone, to die? Why were new mothers told the babies were stillborn? Why were they not "allowed" any human interaction? Why were incurable diseases like cancer not discussed? Why was the norm to keep this from the terminal person? Why did the physician only discuss this with family? Was "hope" more important than truth?

I remember my mother and her nurse friends making a difference. My memory does not recall most of the "behind the scene" plans but I do remember them sneaking back to the baby room to rock the babies until they died. I remember the day they moved the rocking chair back to the baby room. I remember them sneaking the mothers to an area so they could rock their babies until their eyes closed and they could no longer breathe. The nurses would laugh and cry and drink highballs once they had made a slight difference at work. I remember Dena, one of the nurses, pointing her finger at my nose and saying "make a difference."

Lesson Learned: Making a difference has so many meanings. Elders share with their young the joy of what the true meaning is.

26

——wwoorooroom——

CARING NO MATTER WHAT

"Nothing purchased can come close to the renewed sense of gratitude for having family and friends." Courtland Milloy

My mother's cousin was dying of leukemia in the early 60's. I remember her pacing but "probably" not saying a word to him about his illness. She sat by his bedside when everyone told her to "stay out of the room" because you would catch his cancer. He died by himself with his wife and children at home waiting for the phone call.

So have I made a difference? As I reflect over my nursing career I know I have. At the time I did not think about it at all but I remember a small ward full of men that were dying of AIDS in the mid 80's. I would bring them homemade chicken soup and feed these men during my 3-11 shift. All I knew is they were dying with no family or friends by their side. Even the "charge" nurse told me to be careful or I could "catch" this by just feeding them the broth. Of course, I followed the isolation protocol from that era, but numerous nurses said "you never know!!" and I was one of the only nurses that would care for them.

As the years went on and I became a nurse, I remember driving to work and always praying. "Please God, watch over me so I don't kill someone." Her words have always been part of who I am . . . . and God has always watched over me.

Lessons Learned: Nurse angels are many. Some are fortunate to have them as family and friends, to provide them with inside information that will assist them in their journey ahead.

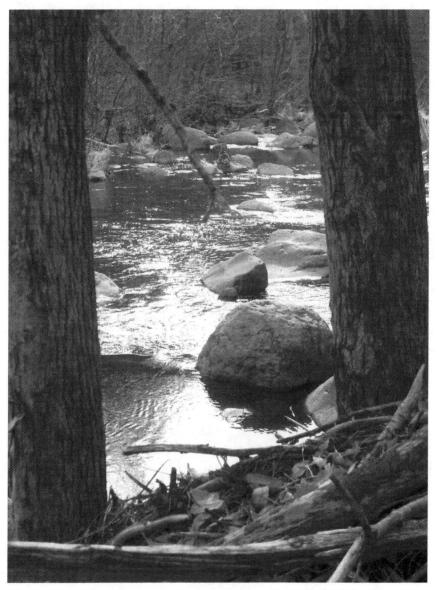

By Amy Govoni

27

TOUCHING THAT ONE PERSON

"You don't have to see the whole staircase, just take the first step." Martin Luther King Jr.

As I reflect back on my nursing career and try to recognize that one special moment in which I knew my presence as a nurse had meaning far beyond what I ever could have imagined happened very early on while I was a nursing student. I had a clinical rotation where I was at a long term care facility for 4 weeks. My assignment was with one patient for most of my time there. I was told in report from the nurse that this gentleman had been very active in the theater in Cleveland and had many friends throughout the community. He had an aneurysm which left him unable to speak, move or breathe on his own. My client had a tracheostomy and it was my job to change his bed, bath him and do his tracheostomy care while I was with him.

In my mind I could never believe that this gentleman could not hear me or understand so every day I come to clinical I would just talk to him telling him everything and anything about my family, school and whatever was going on in my life at the time. In fact, I talked constantly while I was caring for him. Sometimes I thought his eyes would follow me but never did he show any facial expressions, emotion or any movement that would lead me to believe he understood me.

On my last day of clinical at the facility I told my patient that I would miss him and our talks. When it was time to leave I hugged him and told him he was a great listener, which every woman loves, that I was not coming back and it was a pleasure to care for him. Unbelievably when I looked back at him he had a tear streaming down his face. I thought to myself, *Oh my God, he did hear me, and he had to have understood everything I told him.* To validate this I asked him if he would do one last thing for me and that was to give me a smile so I would always remember him and within seconds a big smile come over his face. This was the first and only expression, other than the tear, that I ever got from him. At that moment, I knew I was able to touch people's lives and make a difference far more as a nurse than any other thing I could do.

It has been almost 20 years and I still think of this man often. I tell this story to students I have as a way to make them believe they do and will make a difference in people lives even as a student and they should always embrace the profession they chose and the gift they can give to others.

Lesson learned: Actions and words are important, so don't discount them. Our presence and intention makes such a difference in others' lives, much of which we will never know. Our voices are heard by many that don't seem to be in this world. As we speak, and make the intention of providing comfort and healing to others, know that the impact goes far beyond this world.

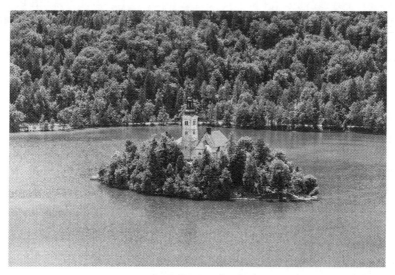

By Bill J. Brodnick

28

THE POWER OF TOUCH

"I think laughter may be a form of courage. As humans we sometimes stand tall and look into the sun and laugh, and I think we are never more brave than when we do that." Linda Ellerbee

I always wanted to be a Candy Striper! Who knew it would happen in an emergency room of a suburban hospital! I remember the family who was waiting to see how their son was after an awful motorcycle accident. I was 16 years old and was horrified by the scene that presented itself to me. Blood everywhere, the screams and grief of a large, Italian family that I could almost feel the pain from. What could I do? A young high school volunteer trying to see if nursing was for me. I remember holding the mom's hand, feeling totally inadequate. But she calmed down and I knew that that touch had made a difference and that I would go on to make more of a difference as a nurse. I will never forget her face and the smile she gave me in all that pain. Something so small, but so powerful that I will never forget it . . .

Lesson learned: Touch is so powerful, we as humans can hardly begin to understand its impact. Keep touching, keep sending loving energy to others. Know it is received with love, even if we don't see the immediate impact. The value goes beyond this world and this one action.

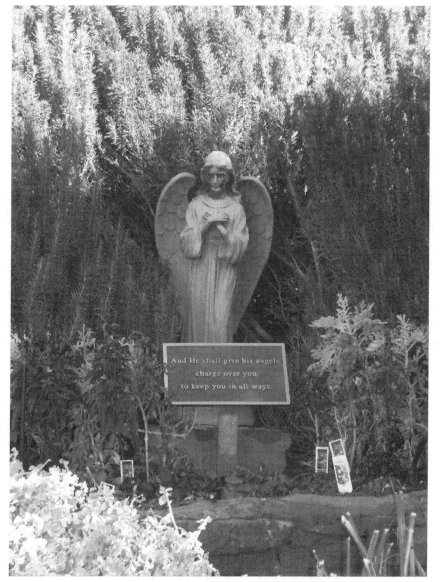

By Amy Govoni

29

THE HONOR OF NURSING OTHERS

"Unless someone like you cares a whole awful lot, nothing is going to get better. It's not." Dr. Seuss

Death has been a constant in my life as a nurse. We all lose people in our lives, but as a nurse, the number of losses through death are immense. We see more death in our short nursing lives than most others see in their entire lives. This woman I will never forget and her husband are medical miracles. She had bone cancer, was on a Stryker Frame that bolted into her head, and sandwiched her body between two framed supports. Pain was always there for her in a degree way past the most you could ever imagine. She smiled through it all; was kind, gentle, warm and respectful no matter what awful treatment we needed to do to her.

Her husband had survived 10 heart attacks, with most needing shocks to get his heart started again. He was so in love with his wife! He felt so guilty that he had been so close to death so many times, and it was his wife, not him, who had to die. He could not have done anything more for her but he kept trying. He held her hand during the most excruciating pain, trying to make her laugh with his jokes.

I was just beginning my nursing career, and I could barely contain my own pain and suffering as I helped this couple towards her imminent death. But they made it feel like I was the most wonderful woman and nurse in the world. They were genuine in their honesty and open with their love and grief. I will never forget their passionate love of life and honor in leaving this world.

Lesson learned: Nothing is what it seems. It is perception that brings either joy or sadness and we have a choice in which one we see and feel. Love transcends many life times. It touches us in so many ways. Is your practice of healing one of love? Do you remember that each day as you start? What a difference that could make for you! Knowing that your love and healing presence will impact everyone you touch that day.

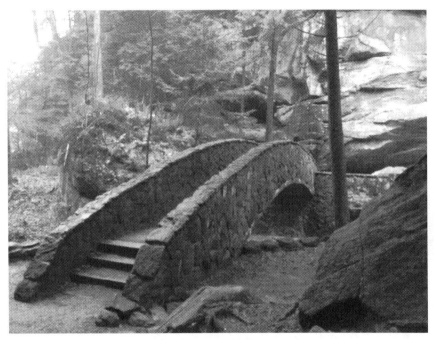

By Jack Ricchiuto

30

USING ONE'S HANDS FOR GOOD

"Most humans look at themselves and how to pull back. They look at how to get by instead of how to thrive and shine. Be the one who shines. Open yourself up for the miracles that surround you. You do this by offering to be the highest Light you can be for yourself and the one of the greatest service for you are here to connect with and be with." From Star Elders

Sadness on the face of a senior citizen, he immediately talks about doctors, pills, diagnoses, physical pain, etc. What is really on his mind is how immensely he misses his wife. He has given up, wants to be with her. The problem is, she is dead . . . he is still alive. I listen, I try to hear what he is not saying. Maybe guilt for surviving when she didn't. Maybe just growing tired of growing old. Maybe just tired of waking up and not recognizing the face or the body that reflects back at him. I just listen . . . and place my hands on his shoulder and knee. My hands and my ears are used most often in this senior living workplace. I have worked hard to listen more carefully, I know I still have a long way to go.

Using my hands was easy. I remember the first time that I felt the tug of compassion so deep that I placed my hands on my babies and soothed them as they wept their infant tears. Now, working in this community of senior citizens, my hands are coming in handy again, using Reiki . . .

Lesson learned: The young, the old, they all want to be touched, understood, and listened to. Energy connects us all and makes us want to share that joy it brings with others.

31

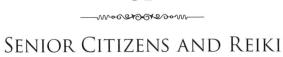

SENIOR CITIZENS AND REIKI

"Plenty of people miss their share of happiness, not because they never found it, but because they didn't stop to enjoy it."
William Feather

"It's called Reiki", she said. That's the first time I heard the word . . . January of 2010 at Yoga Class. "My husband is a Reiki Master-Teacher and it is a form of hand therapy that makes people relax and handle stress and disease better." my teacher said. I was instantly "hooked" and wanted to learn more, lots more. Within 10 months I had become a Reiki Master-Teacher, having achieved all three levels of training and still excited to learn more. On a daily basis, I was given opportunities to practice. My elderly friends were always honest and most often in great pain. They loved to tell me where to place my hands, "Please, my knees hurt!" or, "I feel the warmth all over, even though your hands are on my shoulders!"

My very first resident to let me try my Reiki skills was suffering from the debilitating effects of Parkinson's Disease. She was a "sponge" for my warm hands and my loving intentions would strengthen each time I placed my hands on her. She confided in me, shared secrets that had never been said out loud and our friendship deepened with each day. We cried in each others arms & laughed until our stomachs ached. She told me she was grateful for every day of life, even the days that were full of pain. The Reiki helped her find peace, and her courage strengthened me. Our relationship was a mutual place of understanding and hope.

Lesson Learned: Age, position, none of it matters if you can relieve the suffering of someone else. More opportunities will present themselves to you as you practice.

32

—〰〰◦〜◦◦〜◦〰〰—

BEING GUIDED TO A SPECIAL DOG

"Make every day count. Appreciate every moment and take from those moments everything that you possibly can for you may never be able to experience it again. Talk to people that you have never talked to before, and actually listen." Author Unknown

I woke from a sound sleep as if someone or something was calling me. I knew in every fiber of my being that I needed to get to the animal shelter right away. At this time in my life, it was no small task to get there. I was just returning to driving and was still going for physical therapy treatments for an as yet undiagnosed "dizziness" that had the medical and integrative therapy community baffled. I spent many hours laying on the floor and the couch unable to walk distances without getting dizzy over the previous two years.

My dog family who were with me for 16 years each had transitioned out of their physical bodies and it was time to welcome a new dog into our home. My husband and I had started to look for "the" dog the previous weekend. There were many dogs, all beautiful souls, waiting for their family to come and find them. One dog got my attention while he was digging in the corner of his cage. He was persistent about getting out and really handsome. After a brief discussion about "digger", and knowing that I had reached my walking limit for that visit, we went home.

That morning, I wasn't thinking about "digger" or any of the other dogs in fact. I just knew I needed to get there. On the way to physical therapy I stopped and they weren't open yet. I went on to my appointment and thought I would stop on the way home. I was so tired from physical therapy, I decided that I would go home and rest and go out later. As I came to the street where the animal shelter was, it was as if my car turned itself and in a few minutes I was at the door of the shelter. I went in and was drawn to him like a magnet. The black and white dog, "digger", had been moved to a bigger run and they had trimmed him up a bit and it felt like he was waiting for me. I came to the door of the run and he looked at me and in that moment I knew he was coming home with me.

A quick call to my husband and payment of the shelter fee and "digger" was on his way into our new life. The first stop was to the park for a walk. Yes, I said the park for a walk. It had been two years for me, and he needed to reconnect to me and the earth. These were the first steps in the journey of healing that we both walked together. In that moment, we were both freed from the bonds that held us in an unbalanced state.

The email with a photo of our newest family member was sent out and "digger" was welcomed with open arms and dog cookies and toys. Selecting a noble name for him was essential to reflect the essence of his spirit. His noble name was selected from the Scottish Gaelic, with Birl as his common name.

Birl settled into family life and we learned that which "dog personality" showed up—his cairn terrier or his border collie determined what kind of "activity" he was most likely to demonstrate. When the Border Collie showed up he was busy herding the grandchildren, his boy Matthew and his girl Richelle. When the Carin Terrier showed up, he liked to participate in "ratting" behaviors and we needed to find ways to occupy him so he didn't become "digger".

On our daily walks, we would walk a bit further each day and return to lie on the floor together until the dizziness subsided. Birl and I learned patience and understanding. He just lay with me, quietly while my body calmed down after our walks and I learned how to comfort him when he became anxious and afraid of other dogs and men who smelled like smoke.

There were some other quirks that showed themselves and we used traditional dog training as well as integrative therapies to support Birl's healing. Our world view included the use of the psychic skills and those specific to animal communication. We set up a phone appointment with an animal communicator to see what additional things we could learn about Birl and how to support him in his healing.

The animal communicator started out with an introduction and they immediately said that Birl was really enjoying the oatmeal cookies that were being shared with him at lunch time. The truth was out! When my husband came home at lunch time, he was sharing oatmeal cookies with Birl. Even for us, this was incredible. We learned that Birl had come from a home where there was a more dominant dog that was very aggressive towards him. She also reported that people in the home smoked and the male in the home had been aggressive towards him as well. We also learned that he had left his home and traveled many miles to find me, so we could be together. The moment these words were spoken, I felt their truth. I also knew we had been together before in other lives.

Together we have walked the path of our individual, collective and universal healing. Through meditation, movement, Reiki and other healing modalities Birl has been my constant companion for the last 12 years. He has more gray fur, is slower to move about and his vision and hearing has diminished, yet his noble heart is brighter and clearer and he still loves all of us unconditionally.

Lessons Learned: Our animal angels come to us for many reasons. Teaching, learning and support are some of the top ones. Listen to what your animals are saying to you, without the words of course. They are here to help us in this earthly life. Animals can show us the way to many higher realms.

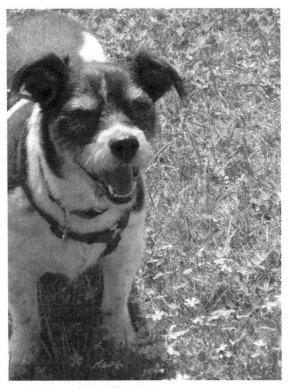

By Michelle Bozeman

33

―――∿⤞⟊⟐⟊⟐⤝∿―――

CAREGIVERS AS HIDDEN PATIENTS

"Expressing gratitude is highly rated by those to whom we share it with. Maybe instead of paying it forward, we could return it backward—thanking all those in our lives who have helped us become who we are today." Janae Bower

My mother had been treated for high blood pressure for several years. She was less than 5 feet in height and 100 pounds in weight, but she had a family history of high blood pressure, heart disease, and stroke. In addition, she smoked cigarettes and was not very active physically. She worked in an office setting outside the home, and in the evenings and on weekends, she liked to participate in craft projects and card games. In the 1970s, while on vacation 1,200 miles from our town, my dad telephoned me to say that my mother had a stroke; then the telephone line went silent. My father had hung up the phone because he was frustrated, bewildered, and upset about what to do. As an only child and nurse, much of the management of mother's care came to me, and so this journey began . . . My mother's stroke caused right-side brain damage that resulted in problems in her movements on the left side of her body and thinking ability. Armed with what now seems like the most primitive collection of treatment options, she received outpatient medical care and physical and occupational therapy after her initial hospitalization. The therapists taught her several exercises that she did on most days with encouragement. She learned to walk again with a cane, with her left leg encased in a heavy metal brace, and she regained some use of her dominant, left hand. As time passed, my father and I realized that my mother did not think or process information in a clear and comprehensive manner. My father would instruct her to not get up and answer the telephone or the door without help. Of course she did both activities when no one was closely watching her, and she fell numerous times, e.g., injuring her foot and breaking her tail bone.

As the years progressed, my mom's stroke affected the entire family; caring for mother became a family affair. Dad enlisted not only my help in caring for her on a daily basis but also that of my husband and two children, who were in grade school at that time. We became closer as a family, but our roles changed. We became the "parents" in watching over my mother. My mother's brother and his wife drove more than 200 miles to visit her almost every month. They provided socialization and stimulation. When the doctor asked my father if he had a nurse coming in to help with her care when she became unable to walk, participate in personal care, or communicate effectively, my father smiled and told him, "The nurse is here when I need her." Mother's sister came and stayed for weeks on end to assist in her daily care and to offer emotional and spiritual support to all of us. My mother's life, her journey here, ended 5 years after her initial stroke.

My life's pathway continues, in that I am passionate about stroke, caregivers and families, caring, and nursing. However, there remains much to be done in providing assistance to family caregivers who are the hidden patients. Oftentimes, caregivers' needs along with their ability to perform self-care are overlooked for the more immediate concerns of their care recipients. Many times my care giving journey felt like a 'test of wills.' However, care giving was also a personal deepening experience where I learned so much and it enriched the lives of all involved in providing that care. May your life's road be well traveled and your journeys unending.

Lessons Learned: Caregivers are hidden patients who deserve the education, tips and compassion just as much as the identified patient. And families . . . they can be the most supportive in the darkest of times.

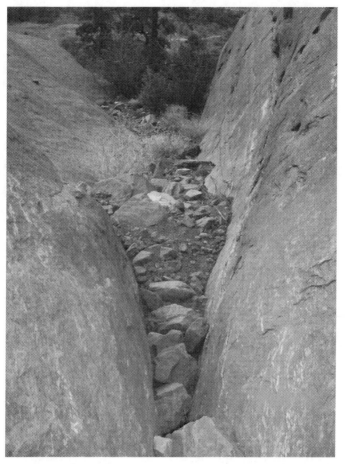

By Amy Govoni

Ending Notes

Now the stories have been told. I hope these stories have sparked an "aha" moment of your own, or an energy filled joyful experience. Take these stories, look at your own and make the changes that give you the endings you want! Our experiences are filled with love, joy, sadness and so many other emotions. You can use them to build the kind of life and stories you want!

If you feel you would like to share your stories with others, remember to email them to me at amygovoni@gmail.com.

I am honored and blessed that you have entered these stories with me! And so it is . . .

Inspiring Books and Web Sites

Reiki Story Resources:

Dyer, Wayne. 2009. *Change Your Thoughts—Change Your Life: Living the Wisdom of the Tao.* Hay House.

Hay, Louise L. 2004. *You Can Heal Your Life.* Hay House, Inc.

Honervogt, Tammara. 2011. *Reiki: Healing and Harmony Through the Hands.* Gaia Books Ltd.

Rand, William. What is Reiki? The International Center for Reiki Research and Reiki in Hospitals. http://www.reiki.org/FAQ/WhatIsReiki.http//www.centerforreikiresearch.org

Ricchiuto, Jack. 2009. *The Stories that Connect Us.* Designing Life Books.

Virtue, Doreen. 1997. *The Lightworker's Way: Awakening Your Spiritual Power to Know and Heal.* Hay House.

Websites:

http://my.clevelandclinic.org/services/hic_reiki_therapy.html
The Cleveland Clinic website describing Reiki and its uses.

www.heartlightyoga.com
HeartLight Yoga Center for Living Well is a unique yoga studio, dedicated to spiritual growth and individualized attention. It is located in Rocky River, Ohio.

www.iarp.org

International Association of Reiki Practitioners website. This site offers information and current status of the Reiki experience. Reiki Practitioners' directory with opportunities for publication in their newsletter and insurance.

http://nccam.nih.gov/health/reiki/introduction.htm

National Center for Complimentary and Alternative Medicine. Information on all kinds of Complimentary and Alternative Medicine or CAM.

www.reiki.org

Reiki website authored by William Rand, a Reiki Master leader in the United States. Much information about Reiki itself, certification, newsletters and other sources can be found here.

http://www.reiki.org/FAQ/WhatIsReiki.http//www.centerforreiki research.org

Rand, William. What is Reiki? The International Center for Reiki Research and Reiki in Hospitals. Good basic information on how Reiki is used in hospitals and research.